Try It Now! CHICKEN SALADS
by Howard Mills

Table of Contents

1. Introduction
2. Spinach Balsamic Chicken Salad with Pomegranate
3. Hong Kong Chinese Chicken Salad
4. Cheddar BBQ Chicken Salad
5. Pepper Flake Thai Chicken Salad
6. Greek Lemon Pepper and Garlic Chicken Salad
7. Poppy Seed Cranberry Pecan Chicken Salad

8. Panera Bread Fuji Apple Chip Chicken Salad

9. Chopped Pineapple-Pecan Chicken Salad

10. Grilled Chopped Chicken Salad with Sriracha and Ginger Sesame

11. Sunflower Honey Mango Chipotle Chicken Salad

12. Black Bean Mango Caribbean Chicken Salad

13. Sour Cream and Avocado Chicken Salad Lettuce Wraps

14. Almond Strawberry and Avocado Spinach Chicken Salad

15. Honey Grilled chicken salad lettuce wraps

16. BLT Rotisserie Chicken Salad Stuffed Avocados
17. Lemon Cranberry Walnut Chicken Salad
18. Grape Roasted Pecan Chicken Salad
19. Peppered Bacon Scallion Chicken Salad
20. Peanut Asian Chopped Chicken Salad
21. Garlic Chili Lime Chicken Salad
22. Toasted Almond Chicken Fajita Salad
23. Cilantro Garlic Chicken Salad
24. Mediterranean Hummus Chicken Salad

25. Curry Chicken Salad with Cashews

26. Mushroom Chicken Salad Cups

27. Pesto Spinach Chicken Salad

28. BONUS 10 Healthy Foods For Women

29. Conclusion

1. Introduction

Hello and welcome to the healthy eating lifestyle. This amazing book contains a compiled list of **26 High Quality** chicken salad recipes that will make your taste buds dance. Each recipe meets restaurant quality standards in the comfort of your own kitchen. These Chicken salad recipes will hold your hand and guide you down the path of healthy living.

Hope you all enjoy these fabulous recipes! "Try It Now CHICKEN SALADS" Volume 2 coming out soon!

2. Spinach Balsamic Chicken Salad with Pomegranate

Spinach Balsamic Chicken Salad with Pomegranate

Servings 2-3

Ingredients:

*Marinade:

- 2 tbsp freshly squeezed lemon juice
- 1 tsp fresh oregano, chopped
- 1 tsp garlic, crushed
- Pinch of salt and pepper to taste

*Salad:

- 6oz baby spinach

- 4 chicken breasts

- Handful of pomegranate arils

- ½ red onion, thinly sliced

- 1 avocado, chopped

*Dressing:

- 1 tbsp balsamic vinegar

- 1 tsp raw honey

- 2 tbsp extra virgin olive oil

- Salt and pepper, to taste

Directions:

1. Combine the marinade ingredients and generously coat the chicken on both sides. Leave it in the fridge for a minimum of two hours, but longer if you can.

2. Place a ridged grill pan on medium-high heat and grill the chicken for about 5 minutes per side, turning once, until cooked through.

3. Whilst the chicken is cooking, combine the spinach, pomegranate arils, red onion and avocado in a big salad bowl.

4. Once the chicken is cooked, transfer to a chopping board, slice and mix in with the salad.

5. In a separate bowl, combine the balsamic vinegar, raw honey, extra virgin olive oil and salt and pepper and drizzle over the salad.

6. Serve.

3. Hong Kong Chinese Chicken Salad

Hong Kong Chinese Chicken Salad

Servings 2-3

Ingredients:

- 1/4 cup mayonnaise

- 1/4 cup plus 2 tablespoons unseasoned rice vinegar

- 3 tablespoons plus 1 1/2 teaspoons sugar

- 1/4 cup soy sauce

- 2 tablespoons toasted sesame oil

- 1 tablespoon Tabasco

- One 1/2-inch piece of fresh ginger, peeled and minced

- 1 small garlic clove, minced

- One 2 1/2-pound rotisserie chicken-meat shredded, skin and bones reserved for stock or discarded

- 3 scallions, thinly sliced

- 2 celery ribs, thinly sliced

- 1 cup unsalted roasted peanuts, coarsely chopped

- 3/4 cup coarsely chopped cilantro

- One small head of romaine, cut into 1/2-inch ribbons

- 1 tablespoon extra-virgin olive oil

- 2 oranges, peeled with a knife and cut into sections

- Lime wedges, for serving

Directions:

1. In a large bowl, whisk the mayonnaise with 1/4 cup of the vinegar, 3 tablespoons of the sugar and the soy sauce, sesame oil, Tabasco, ginger and garlic. Add the chicken, scallions, celery, peanuts and cilantro and toss until coated.

2. In another bowl, toss the romaine with the remaining 2 tablespoons of vinegar, 1 1/2 teaspoons of sugar and the olive oil. Spread the romaine in 4 shallow bowls. Top with the chicken salad and the oranges and serve with lime wedges.

4. Cheddar BBQ Chicken Salad

Cheddar BBQ Chicken Salad

Servings 4

Ingredients:

- 1 tablespoon olive oil

- 2 boneless, skinless thin-sliced chicken breasts

- Kosher salt and freshly ground black pepper, to taste

- 6 cups chopped romaine lettuce

- 1 Roma tomato, diced

- 3/4 cup canned corn kernels, drained

- 3/4 cup canned black beans, drained and rinsed

- 1/4 cup diced red onion

- 1/4 cup shredded Monterey Jack cheese

- 1/2 cup shredded cheddar cheese

- 1/4 cup Ranch dressing

- 1/4 cup BBQ sauce

- 1/4 cup tortilla strips

Directions:

1. Heat olive oil in a medium skillet over medium high heat.

2. Season chicken breasts with salt and pepper, to taste. Add to skillet and cook, flipping once, until cooked through, about 3-4 minutes per side. Let cool before dicing into bite-size pieces.

3. To assemble the salad, place romaine lettuce in a large bowl; top with chicken, tomato, corn, beans, onion and cheeses. Pour Ranch dressing and BBQ sauce on top of the salad and gently toss to combine.

4. Serve immediately, topped with tortilla strips.

5. Pepper Flake Thai Chicken Salad

Pepper Flake Thai Chicken Salad

Servings 2-3

Ingredients:

- 1 tablespoon coconut oil

- 1 small red onion, chopped fine

- 1 teaspoon minced garlic

- 1 pound boneless skinless chicken

- 4 tablespoons lime juice

- 3 tablespoons fish sauce

- 1 inch piece fresh ginger, peeled and grated (or 2 drops Ginger Essential Oil)

- 2 teaspoons red pepper flakes

- Honey, to taste

- 3 tablespoons extra virgin olive oil

- 4 cups shredded napa cabbage

- 1 red pepper, diced

- 3 carrots, grated

- 2 scallions, chopped

- ¼ cup fresh basil, chopped

- ¼ cup fresh cilantro, chopped

- ¼ cup raw cashews, toasted and chopped

Directions:

1. Heat coconut oil over medium high heat. Add onion and garlic and cook for two minutes. Add chicken and saute until browned and the chicken is fully cooked. Allow to cool and shred chicken

2. Make dressing by whisking together lime juice, fish sauce, ginger, and red pepper flakes. Slowly whisk in olive oil until emulsified. Add honey to taste.

3. In a large bowl combine cabbage, red pepper, carrots, scallions, basil, cilantro and chicken. Toss with dressing. Top with cashews and serve.

6. Greek Lemon Pepper and Garlic Chicken Salad

Greek Lemon Pepper and Garlic Chicken Salad

Servings 1-2

Ingredients:

- 1 teaspoon dried oregano

- 1/2 teaspoon garlic powder

- 3/4 teaspoon black pepper, divided

- 1/2 teaspoon salt, divided

- Cooking spray

- 1 pound skinless, boneless chicken breast, cut into 1-inch cubes

- 5 teaspoons fresh lemon juice, divided

- 1 cup plain fat-free yogurt

- 2 teaspoons tahini (sesame-seed paste)

- 1 teaspoon bottled minced garlic

- 8 cups chopped romaine lettuce

- 1 cup peeled chopped English cucumber

- 1 cup grape tomatoes, halved

- 6 pitted kalamata olives, halved

- 1/4 cup (1 ounce) crumbled feta cheese

Directions:

1. Combine oregano, garlic powder, 1/2 teaspoon pepper, and 1/4 teaspoon salt in a bowl. Heat a nonstick skillet over medium-high heat. Coat pan with cooking spray. Add chicken and spice mixture; sauté until chicken is done. Drizzle with 1 tablespoon juice; stir. Remove from pan.

2. Combine remaining 2 teaspoons juice, remaining 1/4 teaspoon salt, remaining 1/4 teaspoon pepper, yogurt, tahini, and garlic in a small bowl; stir well. Combine lettuce, cucumber, tomatoes, and olives. Place 2 1/2 cups of lettuce mixture on each of 4 plates.

Top each serving with 1/2 cup chicken mixture and 1 tablespoon cheese. Drizzle each serving with 3 tablespoons yogurt mixture.

7. Poppy Seed Cranberry Pecan Chicken Salad

Poppy Seed Cranberry Pecan Chicken Salad

Servings 6

Ingredients:

*Dressing

- 1/2 cup mayonnaise
- 1/4 cup sour cream
- 2 tablespoon honey, softened
- 1 tablespoon Dijon mustard
- 1 tablespoon poppy seeds
- salt, to taste

*Salad

- 4 cups cooked, chopped chicken breast (about 2 chicken breasts)

- 1 cup chopped pecans

- 1/2 cup dried cranberries

- 4 green onions, chopped

Directions:

1. In a medium bowl, combine all dressing ingredients. Whisk until well combined. Add salt, to taste.

2. In a large bowl, combine all salad ingredients. Add salad dressing and toss to coat. Add salt, to taste.

8. Panera Bread Fuji Apple Chip Chicken Salad

Panera Bread Fuji Apple Chip Chicken Salad

Servings 4

Ingredients:

- 10 ounces mix of spring mix salad and chopped romaine

- ¼ to ½ red onion, thinly sliced

- 2-3 vine-ripened tomatoes

- 1-2 cooked chicken breast or about 2¼ cups cooked shredded chicken

- 2 cups apple chips

- ¾ cup roasted pecan halves

- ½ cup crumbled Gorgonzola cheese

- ¾ cup Panera Bread Fuji Apple Vinaigrette

Directions:

1. Combine ingredients in a large bowl and evenly divide to serve 4 salads.

9. Chopped Pineapple-Pecan Chicken Salad

Chopped Pineapple-Pecan Chicken Salad

Servings 2-3

Ingredients:

- 3 c. chopped cooked chicken breasts
- 1 c. finely chopped celery
- 2 green onions, sliced (about 3 T.)
- 2 T. finely chopped green pepper
- 1 tsp. salt
- dash of black pepper
- 1/2 c. mayonnaise
- 1/2 c. chopped pecans
- 1 (20 oz.) can of pineapple tidbits, drained
- 2 T. lemon juice

Directions:

1. Combine chicken, celery, green onion, green pepper, salt, black pepper, and mayonnaise in a bowl; mix well. Stir in pecans, pineapple, and lemon juice.

2. Chill for about 30 minutes before serving to allow flavors to meld.

10. Grilled Chopped Chicken Salad with Sriracha and Ginger Sesame

Grilled Chopped Chicken Salad with Sriracha and Ginger Sesame

Servings 2

Ingredients:

*Dressing and Marinade

- 1/4 c low-sodium soy sauce
- 2 Tbsp finely minced ginger
- 3 Tbsp canola oil
- 2 Tbsp hoisin sauce
- 1 Tbsp toasted sesame oil
- 1 tsp Sriracha

- 1/2 tsp salt,

- 1/4 cup red wine vinegar

- 1/4 cup chopped green onions, green and white parts

*Salad

- 2 (9 oz) boneless skinless chicken breasts

- 1 lb napa cabbage, halved lengthwise and thinly sliced crosswise

- 1 1/2 - 2 cups matchstick carrots, or 2 medium carrots cut into matchsticks

- 2/3 cup slivered or sliced almonds, toasted

- 1/2 cup cilantro leaves, chopped

- 3 chopped green onions, green and white parts

- 1 tsp white sesame seeds, toasted

- 1 tsp black sesame seeds (or an additional 1 tsp white, toasted)

Directions:

*Marinade

In a mixing bowl (or 2-cup liquid measuring cup), whisk together soy sauce, ginger, canola oil, hoisin sauce, sesame oil, Sriracha and 1/2 tsp salt (adding more salt to taste as desired). Add chicken breasts to a large resealable bag and add 3 Tbsp of the marinade mixture, reserving remaining. Seal bag and rub marinade over chicken, then transfer chicken to refrigerator and let rest at least 30 minutes, or up to 1 day.

*Dressing

Add red wine vinegar and 1/4 cup chopped green onions to remaining dressing mixture and whisk to blend. Set aside (chill in refrigerator if marinating chicken longer than 1 hour).

*Salad

Heat a grill or grill pan over stove top over medium-high heat. Brush grill lightly with canola or vegetable oil, then place marinated chicken on grill and cook, about 4 minutes per side, or until chicken has cooked through (it should register to 165 degrees in center of chicken when tested with a meat thermometer). Transfer to a cutting board and let rest 10 minutes. Then, cut chicken crosswise into strips about 1/4-inch thick.

To assemble salad:

In a large bowl toss together cabbage, chicken, carrots, almonds, 3 chopped green onions, and cilantro with enough dressing to coat salad. Sprinkle top with sesame seeds and serve.

11. Sunflower Honey Mango Chipotle Chicken Salad

Sunflower Honey Mango Chipotle Chicken Salad

Servings 8

Ingredients:

- 1 Recipe Chipotle Chicken

*Salad

- 1 large head romaine lettuce, chopped (about 8 cups)
- fresh corn kernels from 1 ear of sweet corn
- 1/2 cup grape tomatoes, halved
- 3/4 cup black beans,, drained and rinsed

- 1/2 cucumber peeled, quartered, chopped

- 1 red bell pepper, chopped

- 1 avocado, sliced or chopped

- 1/4 red onion, thinly sliced

*Toppings

- 1/2 cup roasted salted sunflower seeds

- 3/4 cup shredded Monterrey Jack cheese

- tortilla strips or bacon

*Honey Mango Dressing

- 1 1/4 cups chopped ripe mango

- 1/3 cup canola oil

- 2 tablespoons honey

- 1 tablespoon cider vinegar

- 2 tablespoons lime juice

- 1/2 jalapeno seeded, deveined, roughly chopped

- 2 garlic cloves, peeled

- 1/2 teaspoon salt

- 1/4 teaspoon ground cumin

- 1/8 teaspoon pepper

Directions:

1. Honey Mango Dressing: Add all of the ingredients to your blender except the canola oil and chop then puree until smooth. Blend in canola oil. Taste and add additional jalapeno for spicier, honey for sweeter, and/or lime juice for tangier. Chill.

2. To Prepare Chipotle Chicken: Chop or thinly slice cooked chicken.

3. To assemble, toss the chicken, Salad Ingredients, cheese and sunflower seed

together in a large bowl. Garnish individual servings with tortilla strips and drizzle with dressing.

12. Black Bean Mango Caribbean Chicken Salad

Black Bean Mango Caribbean Chicken Salad

Servings 4

Ingredients:

*Caribbean Chicken Salad

- 4 tablespoons reduced sodium soy sauce

- 4 tablespoons extra virgin olive oil

- 2 tablespoons brown sugar (light or dark)

- 2 teaspoons ground ginger

- 4 thin cut chicken breasts* (about 12 ounces)

- 1/2 small red onion, thinly sliced

- 18 ounces chopped romaine lettuce, leafy greens and hearts

- 2 red bell peppers, cored and diced

- 1 cup canned reduced sodium black beans, rinsed and drained

- 15 ounces mandarin oranges in light syrup, drained (or substitute other juicy tropical fruits, such as diced mango or diced pineapple)

- Fresh cilantro, for serving

*Mango Dressing

- 1 large mango*, peeled, pitted and roughly chopped or 1 1/4 cups frozen and thawed mango chunks

- 1/3 cup freshly squeezed lime juice, (about 2 medium size limes, though you may need additional if the limes are not very juicy)

- 1 tablespoon honey

- 1/2 teaspoon ground cumin

- 1/2 teaspoon kosher salt

- 1/4 teaspoon ground coriander

- 1/4 teaspoon cayenne

- 3 tablespoons extra virgin olive oil

Directions:

1. Place the soy sauce, olive oil, brown sugar, and ginger in a gallon-sized ziplock bag, seal tightly pressing out all of the air, and "squish" to combine. Add the chicken, firmly seal the bag again, and move the chicken around gently so that all sides are coated and it lays flat when the bag is on its side. Let marinade for 30 minutes or refrigerate overnight. (If refrigerating overnight, let the chicken stand at room temperature for 30 minutes prior to grilling.) Meanwhile, prepare the dressing and other ingredients.

2. Place the sliced red onions in a small bowl with water. Let sit while you prepare the rest of the salad.

3. Make the dressing: Puree the mango, lime juice, honey, cumin, coriander, and cayenne in your food processor until smooth. With the processor running, drizzle in the olive oil and blend to combine. Taste and adjust seasoning

as desired. Use for salad, then store leftovers in an airtight container in the refrigerator for up to 1 week. Shake well before using.

4. Cook the chicken: Heat a grill pan or an outdoor grill over medium heat. Remove the chicken from the marinade, lightly shake off the excess, and grill for about 2 minutes per side, until cooked through. Remove to plate and let stand for 5 minutes. Cut into bite-sized pieces and set aside.

5. In a large bowl, combine the romaine, red bell pepper, black beans, and red onion. Add the chicken, drizzle with the mango lime dressing. Toss to coat. Scatter the oranges and cilantro over the top, then serve.

13. Sour Cream and Avocado Chicken Salad Lettuce Wraps

Sour Cream and Avocado Chicken Salad Lettuce Wraps

Servings 8

Ingredients:

- 1 ripe avocado, peeled and pitted
- 2 tablespoons sour cream
- 1 tablespoon lime juice
- 2 tablespoons minced fresh cilantro
- 2 tablespoons minced red onion
- 1/2 teaspoon garlic powder
- 2 cooked boneless skinless chicken breasts, cut into 1/2-in cubes (about 2 cups)
- Salt and pepper to taste
- 8-10 butter lettuce leaves

1. In a medium bowl, mash avocado with sour cream and lime juice. Stir in cilantro, onion, garlic powder, and chicken cubes until just combined. Season chicken salad with salt and pepper to taste.

2. Just before serving, fill butter lettuce leaves with chicken salad and serve immediately.

14. Almond Strawberry and Avocado Spinach Chicken Salad

Almond Strawberry and Avocado Spinach Chicken Salad

Servings 3-4

Ingredients:

- ¼ cup extra virgin olive oil

- 1 tablespoon golden balsamic vinegar

- 1 teaspoon sugar

- 1 tablespoon roughly chopped fresh tarragon

- ¼ teaspoon kosher salt

- ¼ teaspoon freshly ground black pepper

- 2 boneless, skinless chicken breasts

- 6 cups loosely packed fresh spinach

- 6-8 large strawberries, hulled and quartered

- 1 avocado, peeled, seeded and cut into chunks

- 3-4 thinly sliced rings of red onion

- ¼ cup feta cheese

- 2 tablespoons sliced almonds

Directions:

1. Whisk the extra virgin olive oil with the balsamic vinegar, sugar, tarragon, kosher salt and freshly ground black pepper in a small bowl until blended.

2. Place the chicken breasts in a shallow bowl and cover with half of the dressing, cover and refrigerate for 30 minutes to 2 hours.

3. Spray a grill pan or 12-inch non-stick pan with cooking spray and heat to medium high. Place the chicken breasts on the hot grill pan. Cook for 3 minutes then flip the chicken breasts. Cook for another 3 minutes, and turn. Reduce the cooking temperature to medium low and cook the chicken for 20-25 minutes

more, turning every 5 minutes or so. Cooking time will depend on the thickness of the chicken, but it will be done when it hits 165 degrees internal temperature. Let the chicken rest for 5 minutes then slice into ¼ inch slices.

4. Arrange the spinach, strawberries and red onion in a bowl. Lightly toss with the remaining dressing. Add the avocado, sliced chicken and top with feta and almond slices. Serve immediately.

15. Honey Grilled chicken salad lettuce wraps

Honey Grilled chicken salad lettuce wraps

Servings 2

Ingredients:

*Dressing

- 1 cup low-fat mayo or Greek yogurt
- 6 teaspoons honey
- 4 teaspoons balsamic vinegar
- 1/8 teaspoon salt
- 1/8 teaspoon pepper

*Salad

- 4 cups diced grilled chicken breasts

- 1/2 cup crushed almonds

- 1/2 cup red grapes, sliced in half

- 1 red apple, diced

- iceberg lettuce pieces

Directions:

1. To make the salad dressing, combine the mayo/yogurt, honey, balsamic vinegar, salt and pepper in a bowl. Whisk together until creamy and well-mixed.

2. To prepare the salad, combine the chicken, almonds, grapes, apple and salad dressing in a bowl using a wooden spoon. Stir until the ingredients are well coated with the dressing. Let chill for 1 hour in the refrigerator before preparing wraps.

3. To prepare wraps, put a large piece of iceberg lettuce on a plate. Spoon a generous portion of chicken salad into the wrap and serve.

4. 16. BLT Rotisserie Chicken Salad Stuffed Avocados

BLT Rotisserie Chicken Salad Stuffed Avocados

Servings 6

Ingredients:

- 12 slices of turkey bacon (3 reds)
- 1½ cups shredded rotisserie chicken (2 reds)
- 2 Roma tomatoes (1 green)
- 1½ cups cottage cheese
- 1 cup finely chopped romaine lettuce (1 green)
- 3 avocados

Directions:

1. Preheat your oven to 400 degrees

2. Lay 12 slices of turkey bacon out on a foil lined baking sheet

3. Bake for 10 minutes, flip, bake for another five minutes, and lay the bacon out over several sheets of paper towels to cool

4. Meanwhile, quarter your tomatoes, scoop out all the pulp and seeds with your fingers, and dice into small chunks

5. Chop the romaine into small pieces

6. In a large bowl, combine the chicken, cottage cheese, romaine, tomatoes, crumbled turkey bacon, and mix together

7. Season to taste with salt and pepper

8. Half your avocados, remove the pits, and season lightly with salt and pepper

9. To serve, scoop ⅙ (approximately) of the chicken salad into each avocado half.

17. Lemon Cranberry Walnut Chicken Salad

Lemon Cranberry Walnut Chicken Salad

Servings 4-6

Ingredients:

- 1/2 cup mayonnaise

- 1/4 cup sour cream or plain Greek

- 1 teaspoons fresh lemon juice

- 1 tablespoon minced flat leaf parsley

- 1/4 teaspoon dried dill

- 3 cups chopped or shredded cooked chicken

- 1/2 cup finely chopped celery or finely chopped apple

- 1/3 cup dried cranberries

- 1/3 cup chopped toasted walnuts, see recipe note directions

- salt and pepper to taste

Directions:

1. In a large bowl, whisk mayonnaise, sour cream or yogurt, lemon juice, parsley, and dill. Add remaining ingredients and stir until combined. Add salt and pepper to taste. Serve chilled on bread or lettuce.

2. To toast walnuts: Place walnuts in a dry skillet over medium heat. Cook, stirring frequently for about 5 minutes, until fragrant and toasted. Watch them carefully so they don't burn. Cool before adding to the chicken salad.

18. Grape Roasted Pecan Chicken Salad

Grape Roasted Pecan Chicken Salad

Servings 4-6

Ingredients:

- 1 pound boiled chicken, cut into ½ inch cubes

- 1 cup chopped celery

- 1 cup red grapes, halved

- ½ cup dried cherries

- ½ cup roasted pecans, chopped

- 1 cup Greek yogurt

- ½ teaspoon salt

- ½ teaspoon ground black pepper

- celery leaves, chopped (optional)

1. Add chopped chicken to a large bowl along with celery, grapes, dried cherries, chopped pecans, Greek yogurt, salt and pepper. If using chopped celery leaves, add these as well. Stir together and serve.

19. Peppered Bacon Scallion Chicken Salad

Peppered Bacon Scallion Chicken Salad

Servings 4

Ingredients:

- 1 lb boneless, skinless chicken breasts

- 8 slices sugar free, nitrate free bacon

- ½ cup of mayo

- 2 scallions (green onions), thinly sliced

- ½ tsp garlic powder

- salt and pepper to taste

Directions:

1. Take your bacon and chop into bite size pieces. Brown and pepper the bacon in a large saute pan over med-hi heat until crisp.

2. Remove bacon from pan and set aside to drain on paper towels, leaving the rendered fat in the pan.

3. Pound the chicken breasts to ½ inch thickness or cut them in half so each piece is ½ inch thick.

4. Turn the heat down to med. Sprinkle the chicken breasts with garlic (if using), salt and pepper and put in the pan with bacon fat. Cook about 2-3 minutes on each side or until the inside is no longer pink.

5. Put the chicken in a large bowl, cover and refrigerate until cool. When the chicken has cooled down, chop roughly into bite size pieces, and in a large bowl, toss together with the bacon, scallions, and mayo. Mix to fully combine.

6. Taste and add salt/pepper if needed. Serve right away.

20. Peanut Asian Chopped Chicken Salad

Peanut Asian Chopped Chicken Salad

Servings 2-3

Ingredients:

- 1 (16 oz) bag of coleslaw mix
- 1 cup cooked chicken
- 1/2 cup chopped bell pepper (any color)
- 1/2 cup cooked edamame
- 1/4 cup chopped fresh cilantro

*Dressing

- 1 tablespoon creamy natural peanut butter
- 2 tablespoons honey

- 2 tablespoons soy sauce

- 2 tablespoons rice vinegar

- 1/2 teaspoon sesame oil (or more to taste)

- 1 tablespoon olive oil

Directions:

1. To make the dressing, add the peanut butter to a microwave-safe measuring cup. Microwave for 15 seconds. Add the rest of the ingredients to the melted peanut butter and whisk until everything is combined. Set aside.

2. Dump the bag of coleslaw into a large bowl. Top with the chicken, bell pepper, edamame, and chopped fresh cilantro. Pour about half of the dressing over the salad and toss well to coat and serve. Add more as needed and store the leftover dressing in the fridge.

21. Garlic Chili Lime Chicken Salad

Garlic Chili Lime Chicken Salad

Servings 4

Ingredients:

- 2 lbs chicken breasts

- 1/2 cup lime juice

- zest of 2 limes

- 2 tablespoons olive oil

- 1/4 cup cilantro roughly chopped

- 2 cloves garlic minced

- 1 tablespoon honey

- 1/2 teaspoon salt

- 1 teaspoon chili powder

*Salad

- Lettuce

- Tomato

- Avocado

- Creamy Avocado Dressing

Directions:

1. Clean the chicken by removing fat, slice the chicken breasts in half lengthwise to make them thinner and easier to cook.

2. In a bowl combine the lime juice, lime zest, olive oil, cilantro, minced garlic, honey, salt, and chili powder. Stir to mix.

3. Add the chicken to the bowl and coat in the marinade. Cover and refrigerate for at least 2 hours to overnight.

4. Heat a large pan over medium heat. Remove the chicken from the marinade. Place in heated pan and allow to cook about 5-7 minutes on each side or until chicken is fully cooked through. Leave in the pan extra time to blacken if desired.

5. Remove the cooked chicken from the pan and set on cutting board to let rest for a couple of minutes before slicing.

6. Assemble the salad, layer the lettuce, chicken, tomato, avocado, and drizzle with the Creamy Avocado Dressing . Or any dressing of your choice.

7. Serve.

22. Toasted Almond Chicken Fajita Salad

Toasted Almond Chicken Fajita Salad

Servings 4-5

Ingredients:

- 4 tablespoons canola oil, divided
- 1/2 cup lime juice
- 2 garlic cloves, minced
- 1 teaspoon ground cumin
- 1 teaspoon dried oregano
- 1 pound boneless skinless chicken breasts, cut into thin strips
- 1 medium onion, cut into thin wedges
- 1 medium sweet red pepper, cut into thin strips
- 2 cans (4 ounces each) chopped green chilies

- 1 cup unblanched almonds, toasted

- Shredded lettuce

- 3 medium tomatoes, cut into wedges

- 1 medium ripe avocado, peeled and sliced

Directions:

1. In a small bowl, combine 2 tablespoons oil, lime juice, garlic, cumin and oregano. Pour half in a large resealable plastic bag; add chicken. Seal bag and turn to coat. Marinate for at least 30 minutes. Cover and refrigerate remaining marinade.

2. In a large skillet, heat remaining oil on medium-high. Saute onion for 2-3 minutes or until crisp-tender.

3. Drain and discard marinade. Add chicken to skillet; stir-fry until meat is no longer pink. Add the red pepper, chilies and reserved marinade; cook 2 minutes or until heated through. Stir in almonds. Serve immediately

over shredded lettuce; top with tomatoes and avocado.

23. Cilantro Garlic Chicken Salad

Cilantro Garlic Chicken Salad

Servings 2

Ingredients:

- 7 oz cooked chicken breast, shredded or diced

- 2 tbsp light mayonnaise

- 1 small scallion, chopped

- 2 tsp lime juice

- 2 tbsp chopped cilantro

- salt and pepper

- pinch garlic powder

- pinch of cumin

- pinch of chile powder

- low sodium chicken broth

Directions:

1. Combine chicken, mayonnaise, scallions, lime juice, and cilantro. Season to taste with salt, pepper, garlic powder, cumin, and chile powder. Add a little chicken broth if chicken seams too dry, 1 tbsp at a time.

2. *To Poach: Cover chicken breast in broth in a small pot, add water if it doesn't cover the chicken. Add salt and pepper, a piece of celery and it's leaves (you could add herbs like parsley, garlic, onion, or whatever you want) and bring to a boil. Reduce to a simmer and cook 5 minutes. Remove from heat, cover tight and let it sit for 15-20 minutes or until thickest part of the breast registers 160 degrees. Chicken will be cooked through. Let it cool and cut into small cubes.

24. Mediterranean Hummus Chicken Salad

Mediterranean Hummus Chicken Salad

Servings 3-4

Ingredients:

- 1 (15 oz) can chickpeas, rinsed & drained
- 3 TBSP water
- 3-4 TBSP lemon juice
- 3 TBSP olive oil
- 1 clove garlic {about 1 tsp minced}
- ½ tsp salt
- ½ tsp paprika
- ¼ tsp cayenne pepper
- 3 cups (12 oz.) cooked chicken, shredded
- ¼ cup grated onion {about ¼ medium onion}

- ½ cup diced bell pepper {about ½ bell pepper}
- ½ cup diced celery {about 2 stalks}

Directions:

1. Add chickpeas, water, lemon juice, olive oil, garlic, salt, paprika, and cayenne pepper to a bowl of a food processor. Process until completely smooth.

2. Transfer to a bowl and stir in shredded chicken and grated onion {along with any juices from onion}. Stir until completely combined. Add in diced bell pepper and celery. Taste and season with additional lemon juice, salt, paprika, and/or cayenne pepper as needed. Serve.

25. Curry Chicken Salad with Cashews

Curry Chicken Salad with Cashews
Servings 2

Ingredients:

- ½ cup mayonnaise
- 1-2 tsp. curry powder
- ½ lime, juiced
- 1-2 Tbsp. fresh cilantro (optional)
- ¼ tsp. salt
- 2 cups cooked chicken, diced
- ½ medium apple, diced
- 2 celery ribs, finely diced
- 2 Tbsp. red onion, finely diced
- ¼ cup raisins

- ¼ cup roasted cashews, roughly chopped

Directions:

1. In a medium bowl mix together the mayonnaise, curry powder, lime juice, cilantro and salt.

2. Next add the cooked chicken, diced apple, celery, and onions until well combine.

3. Fold in the raisins and cashews.

4. Serve in lettuce wraps, on a bed of greens, or on top of cucumber slices.

26. Mushroom Chicken Salad Cups

Mushroom Chicken Salad Cups

Servings 6-12

Ingredients:

- 12 Wonton Cups

- 2 cups shredded, cooked chicken breast, cooled

- 1 cup chopped marinated mushrooms (you can also use canned mushrooms or fresh, sauteed mushrooms)

- 1 cup chopped baby dill pickles

- 1 tub (8 oz.) sour cream

Directions:

1. Preheat oven to 350.

2. Grease a 12-cup cupcake pan with baking spray.

3. Place wonton wrappers in prepared cupcake pan.

4. Bake for 5 to 7 minutes, or until slightly browned.

5. Prepare the chicken salad by combining all ingredients in a medium-size bowl; mix well.

6. Fill baked wonton cups with chicken salad.

7. Serve.

27. Pesto Spinach Chicken Salad

Pesto Spinach Chicken Salad

Servings 2-4

Ingredients:

- 3 cups of chicken, cooked
- 1 cup fresh basil leaves, packed
- 1 cup fresh spinach leaves, packed
- 1 cup Greek yogurt, 7-ounces
- 1/2 cup Parmesan cheese, freshly grated
- 1/4 cup Pine nuts, toasted
- 3 tablespoons olive oil
- 1 garlic clove, crushed
- 1 teaspoon lemon
- 1/4 teaspoon salt

- 1/2 teaspoon pepper

Directions:

1. Chop your chicken into small pieces and add to a large bowl

2. Finely chop your basil and spinach and add it to the chicken

3. Add all the remaining ingredients and stir well to combine.

4. Taste and adjust the seasonings.

5. Serve.

6. To toast the Pine nuts, add them to a small pan over medium-high heat. Once the pan comes up to temperature, they will toast very quickly. Once they are lightly browned and glistening, remove them from the pan to stop the cooking.

28. BONUS 10 Healthy Foods For Women

BONUS - 10 Healthy Foods For Women
& Nutritional Facts.

1. **Eggs** - High source of Protein, Vitamin D, Vitamin B12, Riboflavin.

2. **Greek Yogurt** - Source of Calcium, Vitamin B12, Vitamin B6, Magnesium, Protein.

3. **Fat Free Organic Milk** - Source of Vitamin A & C, Calcium, Protein.

4. **Lean Beef** - Source of Calcium, Protein, Vitamin D, Vitamin B12, Iron, Vitamin B6, Magnesium.

5. **Salmon** - Source of Vitamin A, Calcium, Vitamin B12, Vitamin C, Iron, Vitamin B6, Magnesium.

6. **Beans** - Source of Calcium, Vitamin C, Iron, Vitamin B6, Magnesium.

7. **Nuts** - Source of Calcium, Iron, Vitamin C, Vitamin B6, Magnesium.

8. **Oatmeal** - Source of Vitamin A, Calcium, Vitamin B6, Iron, Magnesium.

9. **Avocado** - Source of Vitamin A, Calcium, Vitamin C, Iron, Vitamin B6, Magnesium.

10. **Broccoli** - Source of Magnesium, Vitamin A, Iron, Vitamin B6, Vitamin C, Calcium.

29. Conclusion

Thank you for trying these wonderful recipes and be on the look out for "Try It Now! CHICKEN SALADS" Volume 2. <u>More High Quality Recipes coming soon.</u>